FOODS THAT LOWER AND MANAGE HIGH BLOOD PRESSURE

Copyright

TABLE OF CONTENTS

SECTION 1

SECTION 2

SECTION 1

What Is High Blood Pressure

The force of blood pressing against the artery walls while the heart pumps blood is known as blood pressure. Blood flows through blood vessels (arteries) at a pressure higher than normal in people with high blood pressure, also referred to as hypertension.

There are two numbers used to assess blood pressure. The pressure in your blood vessels during a heartbeat, known as the systolic pressure, is represented by the first, or top, number. The greater of the two values is the systolic pressure. The force of blood in your arteries when your heart is at rest in between beats is measured by the second, or bottom, number. The bottom number is the lower of the two and is called the diastolic pressure.

Pre-hypertension is defined as blood pressure that falls between 120/80 and 129/89. People with pre-hypertension do not have blood pressure that is as low as they should, but they are also not considered to have high blood pressure. Normal blood pressure is 120/80 or lower. If your blood pressure is 130/80 or higher, it is considered high (stage 1) and 140/90 or higher. If you get a reading of 180/110 or higher more than once, you should seek medical attention immediately. This high reading is known as a "hypertensive crisis."

Understanding High Blood Pressure

Early detection of hypertension is crucial. High blood pressure raises the risk of heart disease, heart failure, and stroke, among other conditions. It is sometimes referred to as the "silent killer" because it may not cause any symptoms. High blood pressure was a primary or contributing factor in over 360,000 fatalities in the US in 2013, according to the Centers for Disease Control and Prevention.

More than 100 million adult Americans—roughly 1 in 3—have excessive blood pressure. However, only 50% of those individuals are able to manage their illness. As people age, they are more likely to acquire high blood pressure, which usually starts in their late 30s or early 40s.However, because of the obesity epidemic, more and more children are also developing high blood pressure.

Average Blood Pressure by Age

	Men	Women
18-39years	119/70mmHg	110/69mmHg
40-59years	124/77mmHg	122/74mmHg
60 + years.	133/69mmHg.	139/68mmHg

Managing High Blood Pressure

Treatment for high blood pressure frequently begins with a change in lifestyle, such as consuming less salt in your food, exercising regularly, quitting smoking, cutting back on alcohol, and losing weight if needed.

Medication is frequently used to decrease blood pressure in addition to lifestyle modifications. Many medication types are available to treat high blood pressure; you and your healthcare practitioner should carefully consider the benefits and dangers of each type of medication. To lower their blood pressure to the target level for therapy, most people take more than one medication.

Within a few days, your blood pressure medicine ought to start acting. It can be difficult to remember to take your medicine because high blood pressure is a chronic medical condition with few or no symptoms. Long-acting, once-daily, or combination medications can help guarantee that prescriptions are taken on time and lessen the stress of taking many medications. When taking medication, you should do so until your doctor instructs you to stop.

Maintaining blood pressure control should be a lifetime endeavor and part of a healthy lifestyle. Your internal organs suffer from high blood pressure, but symptoms do not appear until significant harm has been done.

Controlling your health will help you keep the silent killer under control. It all comes down to knowledge.

SECTION 2

Nutrition and High Blood Pressure

A few little dietary changes, such as cutting back on salt, monitoring portion sizes, and calculating calories, may help you control your blood pressure and cut back on the amount of medicine you use for high blood pressure. Here's how.

Keep a Food Journal

A portion of the population is unaware of their daily caloric intake from food and beverages. They can be under-eating and wondering why they aren't able to reduce their weight.

You can see the truth about your food consumption by keeping a food journal that includes the portion sizes of the things you eat. After that, you can start cutting back to regulate your blood pressure and decrease weight by consuming fewer calories and quantities.

Recognize your alcohol consumption as well. Additionally, drinking alcohol might raise your blood pressure.

Steer clear of salt (Sodium)

Many people have higher blood pressure after eating a diet heavy in sodium. In actuality, you may have better blood pressure control the less sodium you consume.

A teaspoon, or less, of salt is the daily allowance that the American Heart Association advises against unless you have high blood pressure or are at risk (African American, diabetic, kidney illness, or have other conditions). Next, it is advised that you consume 1,500 mg of salt per day. Less than a teaspoon from all of your meals and snacks fits into that.

Understand What to Consume

Conversely, fiber, magnesium, and potassium might aid in blood pressure regulation. Vegetables and fruits are low in sodium and high in fiber, potassium, and magnesium

Stick to whole fruits and vegetables. Juice loses its fiber content, making it less beneficial. Lean meats, poultry, nuts, seeds, and legumes are additional foods that are high in magnesium.

Choose from the following to enhance your intake of natural potassium, magnesium, and fiber:

apples

apricots

bananas

beet greens

broccoli

carrots

collards

green beans

dates

grapes

green peas

kale

lima beans

mangoes

melons

oranges

peaches

pineapples

potatoes

raisins

spinach

squash

strawberries

sweet potatoes

tangerines

tomatoes

tuna

yogurt (fat-free)

Dietary Approaches to Stop Hypertension (DASH).The DASH diet plan emphasizes a diet high in fruits, vegetables, whole grains, fish, poultry, legumes, nuts, and low-fat dairy products. Important minerals including potassium, magnesium, calcium, fiber, and protein are abundant in these foods.

Because the DASH diet is lower in salt and sugar than the average American diet, it can help decrease blood pressure. Desserts, sugary drinks, lipids, red meat, and processed meats are all prohibited on the DASH diet.

As you are undoubtedly aware, a lot of packaged foods might contain hidden salt. However, it's not the only thing to keep an eye on when monitoring your blood pressure.

Sugar

Generally speaking, sugar adds calories with little to no nutritional benefit. However, there are various names for the white substance as well, including agave, sucrose, honey, molasses, brown sugar, turbinado, raw sugar, maple syrup, date sugar, pancake syrup, fruit juice concentrates, and dextrose.

Recall that one teaspoon is equivalent to four to five grams of sugar. The American Heart Association advises adult men to consume nine teaspoons, or 36 grams, per day, whereas the majority of women should not exceed six teaspoons (20 grams). In contrast, the amount of sugar in a can of soda can reach up to 40 grams, or roughly 10 teaspoons.

Nitrates

Most frequently, processed meats like bacon and deli meats are preserved using sodium nitrate. Research has indicated that consuming excessive amounts of these chemicals may raise your risk of cancer and heart disease.

As much as possible, choose fresh, lean meats and seafood over processed foods.

Nutrient-Rich Foods For High Blood Pressure

1. Vegetables and Fruits

** Fruit and vegetables and your blood pressure

Vegetables and fruits are high in fiber, vitamins, and minerals that maintain your body healthy and can help lower blood pressure.

Learn the health benefits of them and how to include more of them in your diet.

** In what ways might fruits and vegetables help lower blood pressure?

A balanced diet that includes fruits and vegetables is crucial for preventing heart disease, stroke, some types of cancer, and osteoporosis (brittle bones).

Potassium, a mineral found in fruits and vegetables, is necessary to keep your body functioning and lowers blood pressure. Consuming fruits and vegetables helps to offset the blood pressure-raising effects of salt, which contains sodium.

They are low in calories and high in fiber, which supports heart health and digestion, and they are rich in many vitamins and minerals that keep your body healthy.

Consume five portions or more each day.

Consume five portions or more of fruits and vegetables each day to help regulate your blood pressure.

What counts as a portion?

A portion is 80g, or a handful.

The sums listed below are considered a portion:

a little salad bowl

three heaping teaspoons of veggies

three heaping tablespoons of pulses, like beans, lentils, or chickpeas one medium-sized fruit, such as an orange, banana, pear, or apple.

two little fruits, such as satsumas, apricots, and plums

a slice of a big fruit, as a mango, pineapple, or melon

three to two teaspoons of grapes or berries

a glass of juice, either fruit or vegetable

a solitary tsp of dehydrated fruit

It is preferable to have some of all of these than none at all.

If eating five times a day sounds difficult, don't give up. Adding two to three portions of fruits and vegetables to your current diet will improve your health, as even a small amount is better than none.

See how eating more fruits and veggies might be simpler than you would think by taking a look at the advice provided below.

Which fruits and veggies are beneficial for reducing blood pressure?

Any type of fruit or vegetable—fresh, dry, frozen, or canned—counts toward your daily intake of five servings. To obtain the whole spectrum of nutrients, choose a variety.

** Canned fruit and vegetables: whenever possible, go for alternatives in natural juices or water instead of syrup, and don't add any sugar or salt.

** Juice and smoothies: regardless of how much you drink, unsweetened fruit juice, vegetable juice, and smoothies are all healthy options, but only in moderation. because the sugar in them can harm your teeth and they are heavy in calories without making you feel full.

** Dried fruit – A 20–30g serving of dried fruit is likewise considered healthy, but because of its high sugar content, it is recommended to consume it solely during meals to prevent tooth decay.

** Pulses: although they only count as one piece, beans, lentils, and peas also count and are among the finest sources of protein and fiber.

** Root vegetables: sweet potatoes and other root vegetables like turnips, parsnips, and swedes count toward your 5-a-day, but potatoes, yams, cassava, and plantains are regarded as starchy foods therefore do not.
**How to increase your intake of fruits and veggies

Including five portions in your day might seem like a chore, but here's how to accomplish it easily and affordably.

**Breakfast:

Top your cereal with a few frozen berries that you can acquire or purchase.

Add dried or stewed fruit to your oatmeal.

In the morning, you can have toast with sliced tomato and mashed banana or avocado

Try making a fruit salad by stirring together yogurt, nuts, and muesli or dried fruit.

You can have a side of grilled tomatoes, mushrooms, or wilted spinach with your eggs for breakfast.

Combine plain yogurt and frozen berries to create a smoothie; all ingredients can be blended together.

** Lunch:

Top sandwiches with salad. Try red peppers with mozzarella cheese, chicken with avocado and salad leaves, or tuna with tomatoes and red onion.

Incorporate more veggies into your soups. Leeks, beans, peas, and mushrooms are terrific choices.

** Dinner

A healthy portion of salad should be added to anything you're eating. To further avoid dressings with a lot of calories, try using balsamic vinegar.

Incorporate additional veggies and pulses into casseroles, stews, and pasta sauces. Vegetables that work well include broccoli, peppers, mushrooms, courgettes, peas, carrots, and kidney beans.

You can use a lot of veggies and lentils in place of some of the meat when creating shepherd's pie or spaghetti Bolognese.

Go for a bean burrito or chili instead of a taco.

Instead than sticking to potatoes, try roasting a variety of vegetables. Squash, sweet potatoes, onions, and carrots make a tasty Sunday roast combo.

** Snack

Throughout the day, a fruit or vegetable snack might act as an appetizer.

A tasty and satisfying milkshake made with bananas and plain yogurt.

Choose oatcakes or crackers with apple slices and peanut butter on top.

Make the most of your produce and fruits.

When purchasing vegetable and fruit meals with sauces, read the labels carefully and make comparisons between the items. They may be high in sugar, salt, and fat.

Consume a wide variety of fruits and vegetables more often. Each will assist to keep your meals interesting and provide your body with all the nutrition and health advantages it needs.

When cooking veggies, try seasoning them with other flavors like garlic, lemon, or orange, rather than salt.

Eat as much fresh fruit and veggie as you can while it's still fresh. If you plan to store them for a long period, opt for frozen or canned vegetables as they tend to lose their nutrients over time.

After cutting veggies, keep them away from heat, light, and air to prevent nutrient loss. When you're ready to cook or consume them, cover and refrigerate; avoid soaking them as the vitamins and minerals may dissolve or wash away.

Vegetables will retain most of their vitamins if you steam them gently rather than boiling or frying them, and use the least amount of water.

2. Whole grains

The Best Whole Grains you should eat for High blood pressure

When controlling your blood pressure, all whole grains are a smart choice. In the end, the type that you prefer and will actually consume is the greatest option, right? Here is a list of some of our favorite whole grains, though, if you'd like to try something different or are unsure of which carbohydrates are whole grains.

** Quinoa

Quinoa is a gluten-free seed that has become very popular because of its excellent nutritional makeup. It is a source of several vital nutrients, including protein, fiber, and magnesium. With an astounding 8 grams of protein per cup, quinoa actually offers more protein than other whole grains! Five grams of protein are included in the same quantity of brown rice, for comparison. Quinoa is an excellent supplement to a diet for controlling blood pressure because it has a low glycemic index. According to an animal study that was published in Nutrients, eating quinoa protein lowers blood pressure and enhances the richness of the gut flora.

Quinoa is also unique in that grain doesn't contain gluten, which makes it a good option for people who have celiac disease or are on a gluten-free diet.

You may increase the amount of quinoa in your diet by preparing meals like a Chicken & Quinoa Casserole

** Oats

Nutrients reports that beta-glucan fiber, a special kind of soluble fiber that functions by forming a gel-like substance in the gut, is one of the many natural nutrients found in this grain that may support healthy blood pressure. It has been demonstrated to lessen the absorption of cholesterol into the bloodstream. Also, a separate Nutrients study found that oat beta-glucan consumption is helpful in reducing high blood pressure

Additional studies that were also published in Nutrients discovered a significant correlation between eating oats and lowering blood pressure and the requirement for anti-hypertensive drugs.

All excellent justifications for preparing a large dish of Old-Fashioned Oatmeal for breakfast.

** Brown Rice

Brown rice is a true whole grain that is high in fiber, vitamins, and minerals because it retains the bran and germ layers, unlike white rice. Its outstanding 3 grams of fiber per 1-cup serving can help with satiety and weight control. It is also DASH diet-approved due to its low sodium content and high potassium, calcium, and magnesium content.

Simple recipes like Salmon Rice Bowl or Easy Brown Rice Pilaf with Spring Vegetables combine whole-grain brown rice with fish and vegetables, which support good blood pressure.

** 100% Whole-Wheat Bread

Another nutrient-dense, heart-healthy food that can help control blood pressure is whole-wheat bread. Because whole-grain flour is created from wheat that contains all three portions of the grain, it provides a natural source of minerals and fiber.

100% whole-wheat bread, like other whole grains, is a good source of potassium, calcium, and magnesium—three minerals that are highlighted in the DASH diet.

Adding additional whole-grain bread to your diet can be accomplished with a straightforward cucumber sandwich. Savor it with a cup of soup or a side salad.

** Buckwheat

Contrary to what its name suggests, buckwheat is a pseudo-grain rather than a kind of wheat. However, because of its same nutritional composition, it's frequently included in the whole-grain group. In addition to being high in minerals and fiber, buckwheat also contains quercetin. According to an American Heart Association study, this plant component has been associated with lowering blood pressure in hypertension patients.

Additionally, rutin, a bioflavonoid that fortifies capillaries and may enhance circulation, is abundant in buckwheat.

According to a study that was published in Frontiers in Nutrition, rutin intake may also help with type 2 diabetes.

Increased consumption of whole-grain foods has numerous health advantages, some of which may be: assisting you in controlling your weight because whole-grain foods tend to prolong feelings of fullness. Raising your potassium level has been associated with a reduction in blood pressure.

Including whole grains in your diet can be a significant step towards lowering your blood pressure if you have high blood pressure and are trying to do so. This is particularly true if your diet is part of a DASH-style balanced diet that supports hypertension. Enjoying a range of whole grains is the greatest option, as they all include vital elements that promote heart health.

You can't go wrong with any of these, even though we're highlighting these five! There are several recipes that embrace healthy grains, such as the robust Quinoa-Black Bean Salad and the sticky Mango Brown Rice. Enjoy the process of trying new things and know that you're providing your body with a variety of nutrients that can help you achieve your blood pressure objectives when you consume whole grains.

3. Reduced fats dairy

Fats, cholesterol and your blood pressure

For the health of your heart, the kind and quantity of fat you eat matter.

Saturated fats in particular cause blood cholesterol levels to rise, which, like high blood pressure, can result in heart disease and stroke.

Watching how much fat you eat will help you maintain your health over time if you have high blood pressure.

How can fat affect your health?

You need some fat in your diet for your body to work properly and to absorb other nutrients from the food you eat.

Fats have a high energy content, and your body stores any fat that is not used as body fat. Eating excessive amounts of fat should be avoided because being overweight increases blood pressure and the risk of heart disease and stroke.

Consuming excessive amounts of fat, particularly saturated fats, also causes your blood cholesterol levels to rise. The liver produces cholesterol, a fatty material, from the fat we ingest. A certain amount of cholesterol is necessary for your body, but too much of it can clog your arteries and narrow them down, reducing the quantity of blood that can pass through them.

This process is called atherosclerosis, and it raises your risk of heart attack and stroke.

Combining high blood pressure and high cholesterol accelerates the development of atherosclerosis, which increases the risk even more, particularly if you smoke or have diabetes. Watching how much fat you eat will help you reduce your chances of major illness and cholesterol.

Saturated fat

Your liver converts the saturated fat in your diet to cholesterol, thus consuming too much of it will increase your cholesterol.

Saturated fat is usually found in foods made with animal products and some plant oils, such as:

pork and red meat

prepared beef products like sausages

cheese cream, ghee, butter, and other dairy products

baked goods including cakes, biscuits, and pastries

chocolate-flavored savory crackers

palm and coconut oils

Try to stay away from meals high in saturated fat when you're shopping. Keep an eye out for goods that have a red traffic light on the label for saturated fat, and check out some more strategies to reduce fat below.

What level of saturated fat is excessive?

Men should consume no more than 30 grams of saturated fat per day, and women should only consume 20 grams.

** Trans fats

Another kind of fat that functions similarly to saturated fat is trans fat. They are found in hydrogenated vegetable oils, which must be disclosed on the label of any food that includes them. Since the majority of individuals in the UK don't consume more than the 5g daily recommended amount, it's more crucial to check the label for saturated fats.

** Unsaturated fats

Selecting unsaturated fats over saturated fats can assist in lowering blood cholesterol levels. Because all fats are high in energy, eating too much of them might still cause you to gain weight. Reducing your total fat intake will also assist to protect your heart.

Which foods are high in unsaturated fats?

Unsaturated fat comes in two varieties: polyunsaturated and monounsaturated. These fats can be found in spreads made with sunflower, rapeseed, and olive oils.

a few nuts and avocados,fatty fish

TIP: Use rapeseed oil instead of olive oil for cooking. Olive oil works great for salad dressings, but it shouldn't be cooked to extremely high temperatures.

Is all cholesterol bad?

Not all blood cholesterol is harmful. To function correctly, the blood must include some cholesterol; nevertheless, too much cholesterol can clog the arteries, resulting in heart disease and stroke.

Cholesterol is carried by the blood in two main forms:

Bad cholesterol" or low density lipoprotein, or LDL. This transports cholesterol to your arteries and throughout your body. It may accumulate within the arterial walls.

High density lipoprotein, or "good cholesterol," known as HDL. This removes extra cholesterol from the arteries and transports it to the liver, where it is metabolized and excreted from the body.

Having high HDL and low LDL cholesterol is the ideal.

Consuming excessive amounts of saturated fat increases your LDL, or "bad," cholesterol; on the other hand, substituting unsaturated fats increases your HDL, or "good," cholesterol.

What level of cholesterol is ideal for you?

A blood test can determine how much cholesterol is in your system.

Use the table as a general guide to what your cholesterol level should be.

Type of cholesterol	What your cholesterol level should be (in millimoles per litre of blood, written as mmol/L)
1.Total cholesterol	Less than 5 mmol/L or less than 4 if you have other health problems
2.LDL cholesterol	Less than 3 mmol/L or less than 2 if you have other health problems

3.HDL cholesterol	More than 1 mmol/L particularly if you have problems that affect your heart and blood vessels
4.Total cholesterol / HDL ratio	Below 4 mmol/L is best

How to lower your cholesterol

A balanced diet is one of the best methods to maintain good cholesterol levels.

Consume a lot of fruits and veggies.

Eat a lot of starchy wholegrain items to fill up.

Consume seafood no less than twice a week. White fish is rich in vitamins and minerals and low in fat. Omega-3 fatty acids, which are unsaturated fats that regulate blood pressure, blood fat levels, and heart and brain function, are abundant in oily fish, including salmon, trout, and mackerel.

Lean meats, poultry, and low-fat dairy products are always preferable to high-fat meats and dairy items.

Swap saturated fats for unsaturated fats.

Swap out full-fat dairy products, butter, ghee, and lard with rapeseed, olive, or sunflower and corn oils.

Include low-saturated-fat foods like beans, almonds, and soy in your diet.

Lowering cholesterol also involves quitting smoking and engaging in physical activity.

Easy cooking techniques to maintain low fat content

The cooking oils we use for frying contribute a portion of the fat we ingest. To help you eat less fat, try these easy tips.

Foods can be stir-fried, grilled, baked, boiled, poached, microwaved, or barbecued in place of being fried.

Use very little oil, and use oils that are high in mono- or polyunsaturated fat.

Try using tomato juice or water when cooking.

Instead of putting oil directly into the saucepan, measure it using a teaspoon or tablespoon, or use an oil spray.

Remove the fat from casseroles, gravies, and sauces.

Before cooking, remove any visible fat from the meat and the skin from the fowl. In order to remove undesirable fat from curries and stews, prepare them the day before and refrigerate them overnight.

Use a trivet while grilling or roasting meat so that the fat may drain off. Substitute unhealthy components with healthier ones; for instance, in recipes calling for cream, use fromage or low-fat yogurt.

4.Nuts and seeds

It's possible that nuts and seeds lower blood pressure. Nuts and seeds that can be consumed as part of a well-balanced diet to decrease blood pressure include:

seeds of pumpkins

Flaxseed

Chia seeds

Pistachios

Walnuts

almonds

Numerous nuts and seeds include a concentrated form of nutrients, such as fiber and arginine, that are crucial for controlling blood pressure. Nitric oxide, a necessary substance for blood vessel relaxation and blood pressure decrease, is produced by the amino acid arginine.

Eating nuts or seeds may help lower blood pressure, according to some research, yet clinical studies had conflicting results.

Researchers speculate that the contradictory findings may be due to clinical trials with nuts or seeds and blood pressure readings being conducted too quickly to detect any possible blood pressure-lowering benefits.

Worldwide, heart-healthy diets include nuts, and scientists have studied one particular kind of nut, walnuts, to determine if eating more of them could lower blood pressure.

Alpha-linolenic acid (ALA), a polyunsaturated omega-3 fatty acid, and several other advantageous plant components are found in higher concentrations in walnuts than in other tree nut varieties.

The topic of whether increasing the amount of walnuts in one's diet could be a helpful tactic to help control blood pressure arises from observational research that correlates diets high in ALA to reduced blood pressure.

For the diet trial, 45 overweight volunteers who were at risk of cardiovascular disease were gathered in the most recent study. The subjects consumed a standard American diet for the first two weeks, with 12 percent of their kilojoules coming from saturated fat.

Following the completion of the lead-in diet, participants were randomized to one of three low-saturated-fat diets.

The diets either included whole walnuts (57 to 99 grams per day),the same amount of ALA from walnuts but without any walnuts consumed, or a diet with an equivalent quantity of oleic acid, a monounsaturated fatty acid found in olive oil, to the amount of ALA from walnuts.

Every diet was maintained for six weeks, with a kilojoule count intended to maintain a steady body weight.

Individuals who consumed walnuts on a regular basis demonstrated the biggest reduction in central blood pressure at the conclusion of the experiment. The pressure on internal organs, such as the heart, is measured by central blood pressure, which is regarded as a significant risk factor for cardiovascular disease.

Similar improvements in blood lipids, including total cholesterol and LDL cholesterol, were seen in all three trial diets.

Eating walnuts lowers blood pressure more than other foods, suggesting that their ALA level is probably not the only factor. This study emphasizes the advantages of consuming entire foods rather than concentrating on specific nutrients because walnuts include a variety of bioactive phenolic compounds in addition to fiber that may help decrease blood pressure.

A heart-healthy diet low in saturated fat may include walnuts as a heart-healthy snack that benefits the heart, brain, and blood pressure

5.Olives

Among the many health advantages of olive tree fruit oil are its ability to decrease blood pressure and other heart disease risk factors.

Olives are one of your five recommended daily foods and are an excellent source of vitamin E and healthy fats.

A review of studies published in 2020 concluded that olive oil can be a helpful component of a blood pressure-lowering diet since it contains nutrients and plant-based substances, such as antioxidant polyphenols and the omega-9 fat oleic acid